REFLEXOLOGY

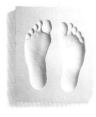

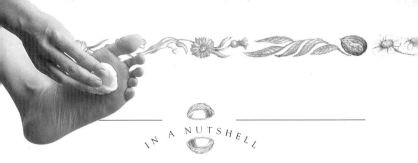

IN A NUTSHELL

REFLEXOLOGY
A STEP-BY-STEP
GUIDE

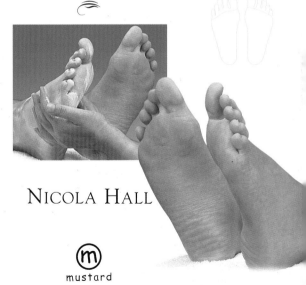

NICOLA HALL

ⓜ
mustard

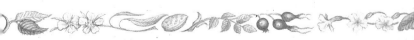

© Element Books Limited 1997

First published in
Great Britain in 1997 by
ELEMENT BOOKS LIMITED
Shaftesbury, Dorset, SP7 9BP

This edition is published and
distributed by Mustard

This edition published 1999
Mustard is an imprint of Parragon

Parragon
Queen Street House
4 Queen Street
Bath BA1 1HE

NOTE FROM THE PUBLISHER
Any information given in this book is
not intended to be taken as a replacement
for medical advice. Any person with
a condition requiring medical attention
should consult a qualified practitioner
or therapist.

Designed and created with
The Bridgewater Book Company Ltd

ELEMENT BOOKS LIMITED
Managing Editor Miranda Spicer
Senior Commissioning Editor Caro Ness
Group Production Director Clare Armstrong

THE BRIDGEWATER BOOK COMPANY
Art Director Peter Bridgewater
Designers Andrew Milne, Jane Lanaway
Page layout Chris Lanaway, Sue Rose
Managing Editor Anne Townley
Picture Research Lynda Marshall
Three dimensional models Mark Jamieson
Photography Ian Parsons, Guy Ryecart
Illustrations Andrew Milne, Andrew Kulman

Editorial consultants
BOOK CREATION SERVICES LTD, LONDON
Series Editor Karen Sullivan

Printed and bound in Portugal

British Library Cataloguing in
Publication data available

Library of Congress Cataloging
in Publication data available

ISBN 1-84164-255-X

Special thanks go to:
Sue Besley, Carly Evans, Julia Holden,
Leon Lawes, Sally-Ann Russell
for help with photography

The Plinth Company Ltd,
Stowmarket, Suffolk
for help with properties

Dwight C Byers, President, Ingham
Publishing, Inc., PO Box 12642, St.
Petersburg, Florida 33733-2642, USA
for permission to use the picture of Eunice
Ingham on page 9

Thorsons, a Division of
HarperCollins*Publishers*,
for permission to use the picture of
Doreen Bayly on page 9

Contents

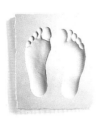

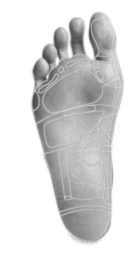

What is reflexology?

REFLEXOLOGY IS A COMPLEMENTARY THERAPY *involving the treatment of various disorders by applying pressure to the feet or hands. Precise areas of the feet and hands relate to particular parts of the body; the whole body can be treated via points on the feet and hands, which are called "reflex areas."*

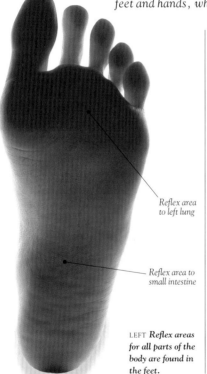

Reflex area to left lung

Reflex area to small intestine

LEFT **Reflex areas for all parts of the body are found in the feet.**

Treatment involves applying pressure to the precise reflex points with the tip of the thumb, or the fingers. The pressure applied is firm but not heavy, and in different parts of the feet or hands different sensations will be felt by the person receiving treatment. The different feelings experienced can be interpreted by the therapist to indicate which parts of the body are working well and which are not. Areas where more discomfort is felt indicate that the corresponding part of the body is more out of balance than those areas where less discomfort is experienced.

Reflexology is also a diagnostic technique – which means it can be used to find out

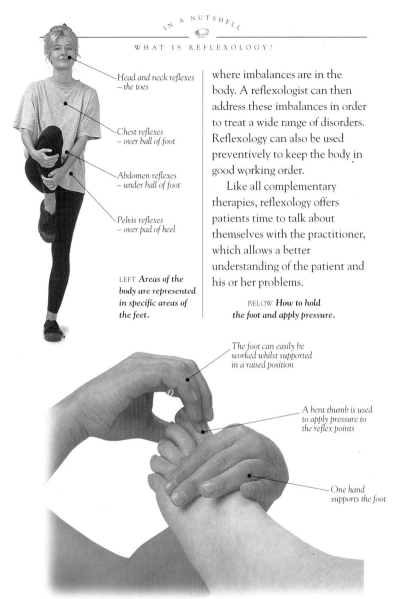

Head and neck reflexes
– the toes

Chest reflexes
– over ball of foot

Abdomen reflexes
– under ball of foot

Pelvis reflexes
– over pad of heel

LEFT **Areas of the
body are represented
in specific areas of
the feet.**

where imbalances are in the
body. A reflexologist can then
address these imbalances in order
to treat a wide range of disorders.
Reflexology can also be used
preventively to keep the body in
good working order.

Like all complementary
therapies, reflexology offers
patients time to talk about
themselves with the practitioner,
which allows a better
understanding of the patient and
his or her problems.

BELOW **How to hold
the foot and apply pressure.**

The foot can easily be
worked whilst supported
in a raised position

A bent thumb is used
to apply pressure to
the reflex points

One hand
supports the foot

A short history

REFLEXOLOGY IS A *modern Western therapy in which pressure is applied to distinct areas of the feet. Although the precise methods of reflexology – and the term itself – are new, similar forms of foot massage therapy have been practiced in different parts of the world over many centuries.*

The Chinese practiced various pressure therapies at least five thousand years ago and these methods probably included a way of working on the feet similar to present-day reflexology. An ancient tomb drawing at Saqqara, dated 2330 B.C., indicates that the ancient Egyptians were also aware of a method of treatment similar to reflexology. Similar methods are also known to have been practiced in India and Japan. Some North American Indian tribes used a version of foot reflex therapy – in particular the Cherokee Indians, who have used the treatment since the seventeenth century and continue to do so today as part of their healing ritual.

3000 B.C.	2300 B.C.	1582	1690	1917
Origins in China	Scene from tomb drawing at Saqqara in Egypt	Book on zone therapy by Dr. Adamus and Dr. A'tatis published in Europe	North American Cherokee Indians used a form of reflexology	Book on zone therapy by Dr. William Fitzgerald and Dr. Edwin Bowers published in the USA – simplified by Dr. Joseph Riley and republished

治

療

In 1582, a European book on zone therapy was published by Dr. Adamus and Dr. A'tatis. Based on the principles outlined in their book and those of earlier writers, Dr. William Fitzgerald, an American ear, nose, and throat specialist at Boston General Hospital, developed his own method of zone therapy, which was published in 1917 with his colleague Dr. Edwin Bowers. Reflexology in its present form developed from Dr. Fitzgerald's zone therapy work and was first brought into general use by an American, Eunice Ingham, in the 1930s. Eunice Ingham devised "The Ingham Method of Compression Massage" which was

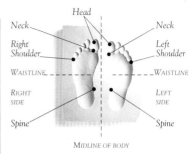

Head
Neck   Neck
Right   Left
Shoulder   Shoulder
WAISTLINE _ _ _ _ _ _ _ _ WAISTLINE
RIGHT   LEFT
SIDE   SIDE
Spine   Spine
MIDLINE OF BODY

ABOVE *Eunice Ingham was the first to chart a map of the body on the feet in 1935.*

introduced to the UK in 1960 by Doreen Bayly, Ingham's student. Bayly also introduced the method to other parts of Europe. It was Ingham who developed and renamed zone therapy reflexology, and she mapped out charts of the feet's reflex zones.

1938	1960	1975	1978	1980
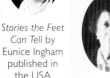 *Stories the Feet Can Tell* by Eunice Ingham published in the USA	Reflexology introduced into the UK by Doreen Bayly	*Reflexology Zone Therapy of the Feet* by Hanne Marquardt published in Germany	*Reflexology Today* by Doreen Bayly published in Great Britain	Clinical studies show that roughly 73% of people treated reported a good result

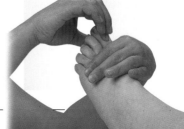

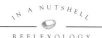
The zone systems

REFLEXOLOGY IS BASED *on the existence of a system of longitudinal (vertical) and transverse (cross) zones or channels in the body. Reflexologists access the body's energy through zones in order to stimulate the body to clear out any congestion which may be causing imbalances.*

LONGITUDINAL ZONES

The ten longitudinal zones, described by Dr. Fitzgerald, extend from the feet up the legs and up the body to the head, and down the arms to the hands. These zones could also be described in reverse as running from the hands up the arms to the head, and then down the body to the feet. There are five zones on the right side of the body and five zones on the left side of the body, with zone 1 connecting the big toe and the thumb, zone 2 the second toe and second finger, zone 3 the third toe and third finger, zone 4 the fourth toe and fourth finger, and zone 5 the little toe and little finger. The zones are segments through the body which are at equal width at any section of the body.

Within the zones, there is a flow of energy which runs through every part of the body situated within the same zone. The zones extend to the feet and hands, so reflex areas relating to the different body parts will be found in the same zones of the feet and hands. From this it is easy to map out the areas of the body which correspond to the appropriate reflex points on the feet and hands.

THE LONGITUDINAL ZONES IN THE FEET

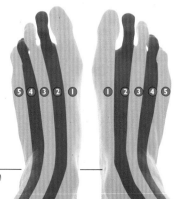

THE LONGITUDINAL AND
TRANSVERSE ZONES OF THE BODY

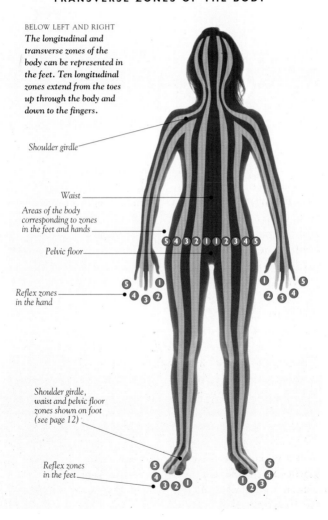

BELOW LEFT AND RIGHT
The longitudinal and transverse zones of the body can be represented in the feet. Ten longitudinal zones extend from the toes up through the body and down to the fingers.

Shoulder girdle

Waist

Areas of the body corresponding to zones in the feet and hands

Pelvic floor

Reflex zones in the hand

Shoulder girdle, waist and pelvic floor zones shown on foot (see page 12)

Reflex zones in the feet

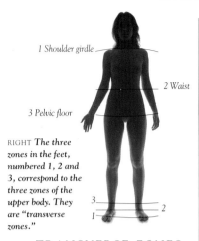

1 Shoulder girdle

2 Waist

3 Pelvic floor

3
2
1

RIGHT *The three zones in the feet, numbered 1, 2 and 3, correspond to the three zones of the upper body. They are "transverse zones."*

TRANSVERSE ZONES

Transverse zones are also identified in the feet, and these were first described by Hanne Marquardt, a German practitioner. These zones or areas show how three levels in the body, running horizontally, can be found in the feet – marked by the foot bones. The three levels are the shoulder girdle, waist, and pelvic floor. There are 26 bones in the feet: 14 phalanges, found in the toes, 5 metatarsals below these, and then 7 tarsals. The level of the shoulder girdle is where the phalanges meet the metatarsal bones; the level of the waist is about halfway down the foot, where the metatarsals meet the tarsal bones; the level of the pelvic floor is an imaginary line across the tarsal bones between the ankle bones. These transverse areas help to divide the foot to identify more clearly which parts of the foot relate to which parts of the body.

MERIDIANS

Some authorities claim that reflexology is working not on the longitudinal zones but on meridians found in the body, since these extend to the feet and hands. Meridians are used as a basis for much Chinese medicine; they are channels which run through and contain the energy of the body. The twelve meridians (used in acupuncture, acupressure, and other systems) are not the same as the longitudinal zones but much of the ideology is similar.

Acupuncture meridians are fine lines which run through the body in a clearly defined system. Some reflexologists will work on the acupuncture points during treatment. It remains to be proven whether or not reflexologists and acupuncturists are working on the same points.

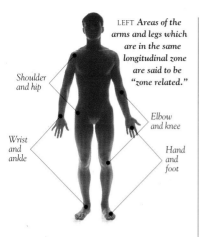

LEFT *Areas of the arms and legs which are in the same longitudinal zone are said to be "zone related."*

Shoulder and hip

Elbow and knee

Wrist and ankle

Hand and foot

ZONE-RELATED AREAS

Since the ten longitudinal zones pass through the body and down the arms and legs, the arms and legs are said to be "zone-related" with a special relationship existing between the shoulder and the hip; the elbow and the knee; the wrist and the ankle; the hand and the foot.

The areas between the joints can also be related; i.e., the upper arm related to the upper leg and the forearm to the lower leg. There is a link between parts on the same side of the body: the right elbow is related to the right knee, and the left wrist is related to the left ankle.

In addition to working directly on the affected area, a reflexologist can work on a zone-related area, which is particularly helpful when a body part is inaccessible or extremely painful. For example, if the patient suffered from a very painful right knee, the right elbow could be massaged using reflexology pressure techniques; for a broken left ankle, the left wrist could be massaged to encourage the healing process.

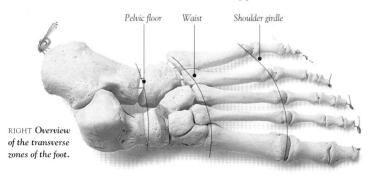

Pelvic floor   Waist   Shoulder girdle

RIGHT **Overview of the transverse zones of the foot.**

How does reflexology work?

LIKE MANY COMPLEMENTARY *therapies, reflexology has no proven scientific theory, other than the fact that nerve endings (there are 70,000 on the sole of each foot) are stimulated. Most reflexologists believe that by working on reflex areas, we are able to balance the energy flow within the longitudinal zones of the body and so help correct body functioning.*

LIFESTYLES

One of the most common reasons for ill health is stress – the effects of the

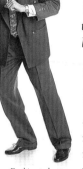

Rushing to keep appointments

pressures of daily life on our bodies, and the other demands placed upon the body, such as dealing with pollution, additives and pesticides in our food, and city living.

We are all affected by stress in different ways, and many develop a variety of physical problems as a result, including headaches and migraines,

tension in the neck, backache, digestive disorders, a weakened immune system, high blood pressure, skin conditions, and frequent colds and infections.

Working while eating and being at the beck and call of mobile telephones

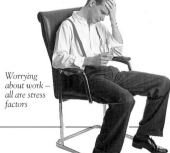

Worrying about work – all are stress factors

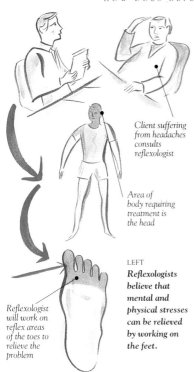

Client suffering from headaches consults reflexologist

Area of body requiring treatment is the head

Reflexologist will work on reflex areas of the toes to relieve the problem

LEFT
Reflexologists believe that mental and physical stresses can be relieved by working on the feet.

body as a whole, not as a group of symptoms – and can help both physically and mentally. Symptoms that have occurred in the body due to stress can be eased, and the balancing effect of the treatment improves our overall health, by dealing with the root cause of the symptoms, not just the symptoms themselves. When we feel better physically, we feel better psychologically, and an improved sense of well-being can also reduce stress levels and prevent further illness. After treatment you will feel calmer, more peaceful, and more positive, and therefore able to cope with stress and any related health conditions.

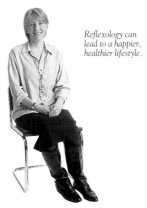

Reflexology can lead to a happier, healthier lifestyle.

BETTER LIFESTYLES

Although reflexology cannot prevent the stresses that occur in everyday life, it can help us to cope better with the stress and be more relaxed. One of the most important benefits of reflexology is relaxation.

The treatment is an holistic one – which means it treats the

The treatment

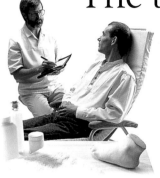

BEFORE TREATMENT COMMENCES *a detailed medical history will be taken. Your practitioner will take a full case history – that is, everything there is to know about you and your health, from your physical symptoms and sleeping habits to all aspects of your lifestyle, and your emotional condition. This allows your therapist to focus on the kind of treatment which will be appropriate to you as an individual, and to determine whether it is appropriate for reflexology treatment to be given.*

ABOVE **A detailed medical history will be taken by the practitioner before treatment starts.**

You will be seated in a reclining position so that you are comfortable – with your back, neck, and legs well supported, and with the feet raised so that the practitioner can comfortably work on them. Unless it is impossible for some reason, your reflexologist will treat your feet.

An examination of the feet is the first step, and then your practitioner usually wipes them with moist wipes to remove superficial dirt or to cool the feet on a hot day. Signs of hard skin, corns, cracks between the toes,

an area of infection such as a verruca, and nail problems will all be identified.

A small amount of talcum powder may be massaged onto the feet. Talc is often used for treatment as it will absorb moisture if the feet are a bit wet, and make them smooth if they are very dry. Some practitioners may use oils instead, but this is not always advised. General massage will be given to the feet to enable you to get used to the practitioner's touch and also to help you to relax.

Once you are used to having your feet worked, the practitioner will explain how the treatment is to be given; reassurance will be offered if you are concerned about experiencing any pain.

Reflexology is not painful; tender areas are treated gently and the feeling tends to be soothing rather than sore. A precise soothing technique *(see pages 26–7)* will then be applied to all of the reflex points in both feet.

RELAXING THROUGH REFLEXOLOGY

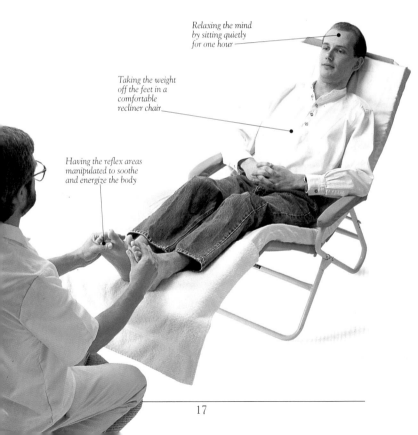

Relaxing the mind by sitting quietly for one hour

Taking the weight off the feet in a comfortable recliner chair

Having the reflex areas manipulated to soothe and energize the body

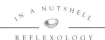
How treatment is given

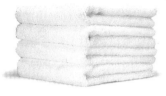

ABOVE **Towels are used to cushion the feet during treatment.**

MOST PARTS OF THE *body are duplicated on both the left and right sides of the body, and the reflex points for these body parts will appear in roughly the same position on both feet. Some parts of the body are found on just one side – for example, the heart –* and therefore will be represented on only one foot, in this case the left. *Reflex areas are found on the soles, sides and tops of feet, and every part of the feet has a corresponding part of the body.*

There is a map of the body mirrored in the shape of the hands and feet, divided by longitudinal and transverse zones (*see pages 10–12*). Each body part has a corresponding reflex area in the feet and hands.

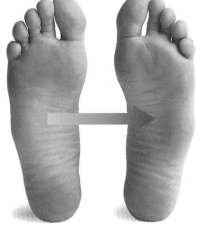

RIGHT **Treatment will usually be given to all areas of the right foot and then all areas of the left foot.**

Treatment is often given to the reflex areas in the right foot first, and then the left, although this can differ between practitioners. Having worked on both feet, reflex areas to affect part of the body are then given extra attention. In this instance, both feet may be worked simultaneously; for example, the kidney reflexes on both feet may be stimulated for best effect.

WHAT DOES IT FEEL LIKE?

1 Different sensations will be felt according to the personal characteristics of each patient. The greater the degree of tenderness, the more out of balance the corresponding part of the body.

2 In some areas, pressure will be felt but no discomfort.

3 In some areas, pressure may feel slightly uncomfortable.

4 In some areas, pressure may cause a sharp twinge, almost as if a nail were being stuck into the foot (this is a fleeting sensation, and is instantly relieved by your practitioner).

Reflex to head

Reflex to thyroid gland

LEFT *The feet are always supported while treatment is given. The whole foot is worked first, then the areas that need special attention.*

Reflex to kidney

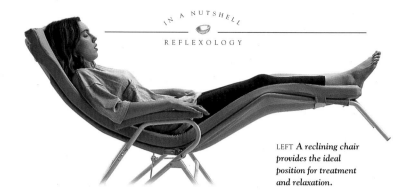

LEFT *A reclining chair provides the ideal position for treatment and relaxation.*

LENGTH OF TREATMENT

A treatment session will last about one hour, and will be given at weekly intervals. Although improvement may occur after just one treatment, it is important to have a course of at least three treatments to ensure that the improvements achieved are maintained. It will become evident after three treatments whether or not your particular condition will respond to reflexology. Some people like to return every six weeks to two months for a "top up" to restore balance to the body.

LENGTH OF TREATMENT

• A treatment session lasts about one hour.

• Expect to have at least three treatments, usually one per week.

• A course of four to six treatments is usually required.

• The interval between treatments can be extended as improvements occur.

• Regular treatment can continue to maintain improvements and prevent further imbalances.

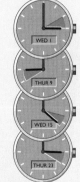

Moist wipes are used to clean and refresh the feet

Any foot infections are identified

LEFT *The feet may be wiped over before treatment to remove any dirt.*

Reactions to treatment can occur as the body begins to clear out toxins – slight nausea and mild diarrhea may be experienced, but no reaction should be strong enough to be disturbing. Symptoms like these are usually an encouraging sign because they indicate that the treatment is working.

POSSIBLE REACTIONS EXPERIENCED

- Cold-like symptoms such as a running nose, as catarrh and sinus congestion are cleared

- A cough, as mucus is cleared from the lungs and respiratory passages

- More frequent emptying of the bladder

- More frequent emptying of the bowels

- Flatulence

- Headache

- Increased sweating

- Skin rash – some skin conditions may get worse before they get better

- Yawning

- Tiredness

- Increased energy

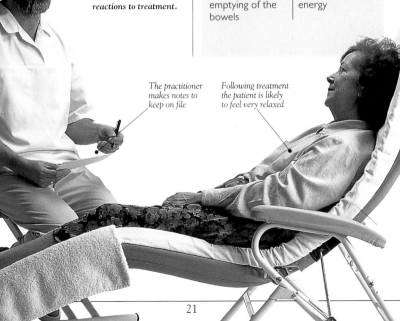

BELOW *The practitioner will record the findings from the treatment and advise of any possible reactions to treatment.*

The practitioner makes notes to keep on file

Following treatment the patient is likely to feel very relaxed

21

THE RIGHT FOOT

Each precise area
of the right foot is
directly related to a
specific part of the
right side of the body.

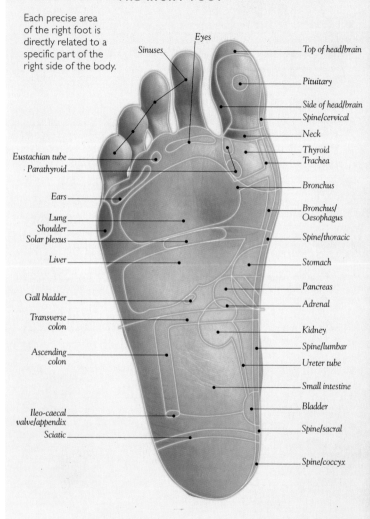

Eyes

Sinuses

Eustachian tube
Parathyroid

Ears

Lung
Shoulder
Solar plexus

Liver

Gall bladder

Transverse
colon

Ascending
colon

Ileo-caecal
valve/appendix
Sciatic

Top of head/brain

Pituitary

Side of head/brain
Spine/cervical

Neck

Thyroid
Trachea

Bronchus

Bronchus/
Oesophagus

Spine/thoracic

Stomach

Pancreas

Adrenal

Kidney

Spine/lumbar
Ureter tube

Small intestine

Bladder

Spine/sacral

Spine/coccyx

THE LEFT FOOT

Each precise area of the left foot is directly related to a specific part of the left side of the body.

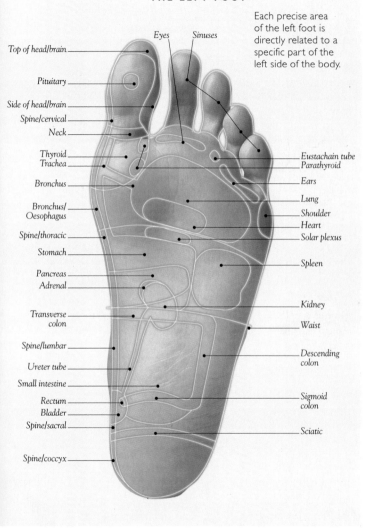

Eyes
Sinuses
Top of head/brain
Pituitary
Side of head/brain
Spine/cervical
Neck
Thyroid
Trachea
Bronchus
Bronchus/Oesophagus
Spine/thoracic
Stomach
Pancreas
Adrenal
Transverse colon
Spine/lumbar
Ureter tube
Small intestine
Rectum
Bladder
Spine/sacral
Spine/coccyx

Eustachain tube
Parathyroid
Ears
Lung
Shoulder
Heart
Solar plexus
Spleen
Kidney
Waist
Descending colon
Sigmoid colon
Sciatic

THE SIDES OF THE FEET

The reproductive
reflexes are mainly
located in the sides
of the feet and
the ankles.

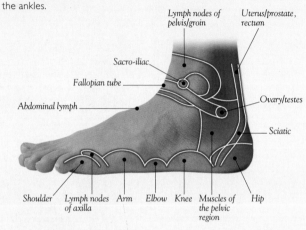

Lymph nodes of pelvis/groin

Uterus/prostate, rectum

Sacro-iliac

Fallopian tube

Abdominal lymph

Ovary/testes

Sciatic

Shoulder   Lymph nodes   Arm   Elbow   Knee   Muscles of   Hip
            of axilla   the pelvic
                                                   region

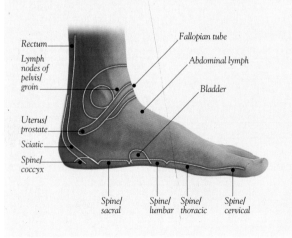

Rectum

Lymph
nodes of
pelvis/
groin

Fallopian tube

Abdominal lymph

Bladder

Uterus/
prostate

Sciatic

Spine/
coccyx

Spine/   Spine/   Spine/   Spine/
sacral   lumbar   thoracic   cervical

THE TOPS OF THE FEET

The reflexes of the lymphatic system are mainly located over the tops of the feet.

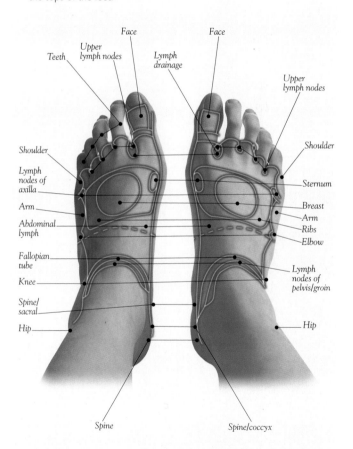

Face

Face

Teeth

Upper lymph nodes

Lymph drainage

Upper lymph nodes

Shoulder

Shoulder

Lymph nodes of axilla

Sternum

Arm

Breast

Abdominal lymph

Arm

Ribs

Elbow

Fallopian tube

Knee

Lymph nodes of pelvis/groin

Spine/sacral

Hip

Hip

Spine

Spine/coccyx

How to hold the foot

BOTH HANDS ARE USED *by the reflexologist, with the thumb or fingers of one hand applying the massage and the other hand supporting the area being worked on.*

Pressure is applied using the side of the tip of the thumb. As pressure is applied, the fingernail is pressed back against the thumb to avoid pressing the nail into the foot. Pressure is held on each point for just a moment before moving to the next point.

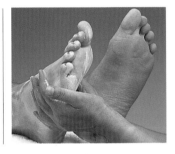

Both hands are in contact with the feet throughout the treatment

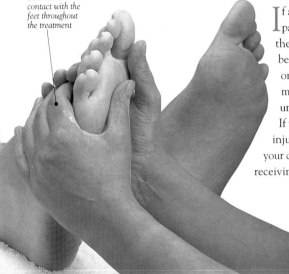

If a reflex point shows particular sensitivity, then the pressure will be reduced but held on the point for a moment or so longer until the pain eases. If you have a serious injury, you must see your doctor before receiving treatment.

LEFT *The foot is supported while it is examined.*

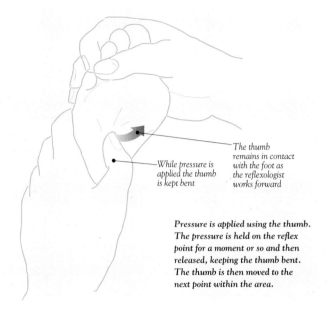

The thumb remains in contact with the foot as the reflexologist works forward

While pressure is applied the thumb is kept bent

Pressure is applied using the thumb. The pressure is held on the reflex point for a moment or so and then released, keeping the thumb bent. The thumb is then moved to the next point within the area.

The thumb moves in a forward direction to work the reflex points within an area. The thumb is held bent at all times. The pressure is applied to a reflex point and then released; the thumb is lifted just off the point and then the next, adjacent point is massaged. As much as possible, the thumb should be kept in contact with the foot, creating a smooth technique, not a prodding action.

In certain areas, the presence of crystal-like deposits may be felt just beneath the skin surface. These indicate imbalances and can be worked on by carefully rotating the tip of the thumb over the area, which may help to disperse the deposits.

Always hold the foot firmly but gently. You may be reluctant to apply strong pressure as you work, but with practice you will learn to be firm without being rough or causing pain.

Step-by-step treatment guide

*BELOW **The whole body area can be worked on during a single treatment.***

A FULL TREATMENT *will involve working all of the areas on the right foot, and then all of the areas on the left foot – starting with the toes, and working each section of the sole of the foot, and then the sides and top of the foot.*

Reflexes to the chest are on the sole of the foot, in the ball area

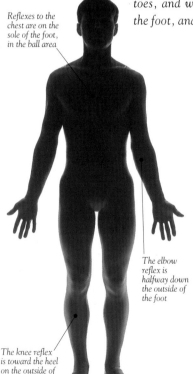

The elbow reflex is halfway down the outside of the foot

The knee reflex is toward the heel on the outside of the foot

HEAD AND NECK

The reflex areas for the parts of the head and neck are found within the toe areas.

SPINE

The reflex area for the spine is found down the inner border of both feet.

CHEST

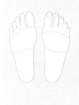

The reflex areas for the parts of the chest are found between the levels of the shoulder girdle and the diaphragm on both feet.

ABDOMEN

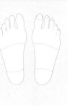

The reflex areas for the parts of the abdomen are found below the level of the diaphragm to just above the pad of the heel on both feet.

PELVIS

The reflex areas for the parts of the pelvis are found just above and over the pad of the heel and on the sides of the feet near the ankle bones.

LIMBS

The reflex areas for the limbs are found on the outer side of the feet.

REPRODUCTIVE GLANDS

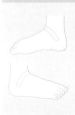

The reflex areas for the reproductive glands are found on the sides of the feet near and over the ankles.

LYMPHATIC SYSTEM

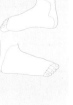

The reflex areas for the lymphatics and breast are found on the top of the feet.

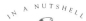

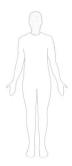

The head and neck

THE REFLEX AREAS (reflexes) for the head and neck areas are found in the areas of the toes in both feet and, in addition, the whole of the head can be presented within the big toe area on each foot.

1 On the sole of the big toe, the top of the toe represents the top of the head and brain, the outer side represents the outer side of the head and brain, and the base represents the back of the head and brain. The reflex to the pituitary gland is near the center of the pad of the big toe.

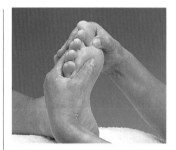

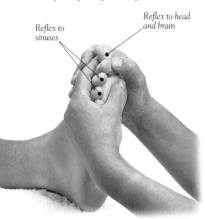

Reflex to sinuses

Reflex to head and brain

2 Around the base of the big toe, just above where it joins the foot, is the reflex to the neck. The base of the big toe represents the back of the neck. The side of the base of the big toe represents the seventh cervical, or last, vertebra in the neck, where many of the nerves of the arm and hand pass.

LEFT *The toes are the site of the head and neck reflexes, including the sinuses.*

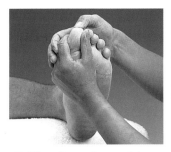

3 The reflex to the top of the head and the top of the brain is found just behind the big toe nail.

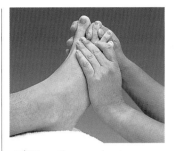

5 The reflexes to the sinuses are found up the back and the sides of the toes.

The face reflex

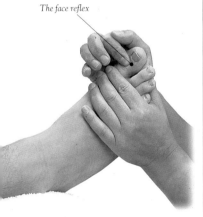

4 On the front of the big toe is the face reflex. The upper aspects of the other toes also relate to the face – in particular the teeth and gums. At the base of the big toe, just above where it joins the foot, is a neck reflex.

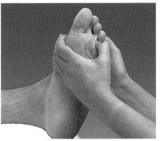

6 The reflex to the eye is found just beneath where the second and third toes join the soles of the feet. The reflex to the ear is found just beneath where the fourth and fifth toes join the soles of the feet. The reflex to the Eustachian tube (that connects ear to throat) is found between the eye and ear reflexes.

The spine

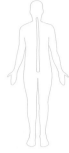

THE REFLEX to the spine is found down the inner side of the foot in both feet, following the bony arch of the foot from the side of the big toe to the back of the heel. Along the spine reflex are reflexes for the upper part of the spine (cervical or neck region), reflexes for the middle or thoracic region, reflexes for the lower (lumbar) region, and reflexes for the tailbone and sacrum (bottom of the spine). Treatment begins at the top of the reflex area to the spine, and works down the inner edge of the heel.

1 The inside of each foot is the area which corresponds to the parts of the spine. The natural curve of the foot area mirrors the shape of the spine, and so the upper, middle, and lower regions of the spine and the tailbone can easily be "plotted" along the reflex.

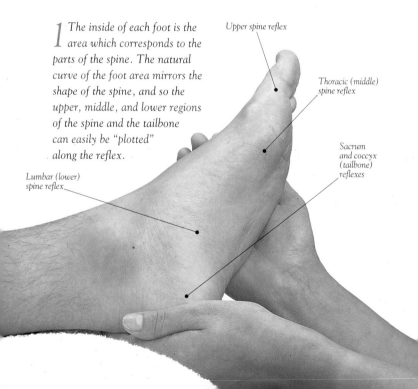

Upper spine reflex

Thoracic (middle) spine reflex

Sacrum and coccyx (tailbone) reflexes

Lumbar (lower) spine reflex

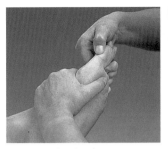

2 The reflex for the upper part of the spine, the cervical or neck region, is located along the edge of the big toe.

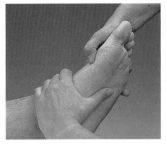

3 The reflex for the thoracic (middle) region of the spine can be found along the edge of the first metatarsal bone (see page 12), down to waist level.

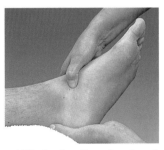

4 The lumbar (lower) region of the spine is represented from below waist level along the tarsal bones (see page 12), following the bony arch along the inner side of the foot, and ending at a point approximately level with the inner ankle bone. The reflex for the bladder is just below the lumbar region on the inside of each foot.

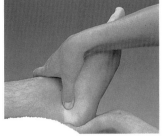

5 The sacrum and coccyx (tailbone) at the base of the spine are located along the tarsal bones, just before the back of the heel. The sciatic reflex – the sciatic nerve itself – travels down both sides of the leg, and across the heel like a stirrup, making this area a particularly sensitive part of the foot.

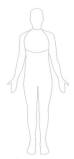

The chest

THE REFLEXES *to the chest area can be found on the sole of the foot in the area between the level of the shoulder girdle (roughly the base of the toes), and the diaphragm (or waist) area, which sits just below the ball of each foot, and in a similar area on the top of the foot.*

The chest area on the foot contains reflexes to the following: parts of the respiratory system, including the trachea (windpipe), bronchi (air passages) and lungs; the heart; the esophagus (down which food travels from the mouth to the stomach); the thyroid and the parathyroid glands (see below); the ribs and sternum. The chest area of the foot is also the site of reflex points for important structures that lead to the digestive system, and contains the nerve that controls the diaphragm.

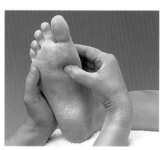

1 *The reflexes for the thyroid gland are on the outer edge of the ball of the big toe on both feet.*

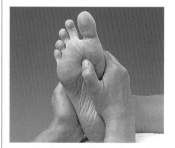

2 *The four small parathyroid glands affect levels of calcium and phosphorus in the body. The lower parathyroid reflexes are located at the lower outer edge of the ball of the big toe.*

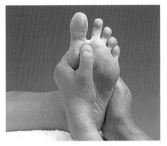

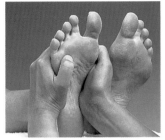

3 The upper parathyroid reflexes can be found at the upper outer edge of the ball of the big toe on each foot.

4 The reflexes to the lung are found over the ball of the foot. The reflex to the bronchi extends across the lower part of the ball of the big toe into the lung area – from the reflex to the trachea, which is found down the inner edge of the sole of the foot from the base of the big toe to near the base of the ball of the big toe.

Thumb working on the heart reflex on the left foot

5 The reflex to the esophagus overlaps that of the trachea but extends down to diaphragm level on both feet. The reflex to the heart is found only on the left foot, in an area just above the level of the diaphragm.

The abdomen

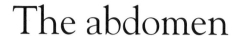

THE REFLEX AREA *for the abdomen is between the levels of the diaphragm (just below the ball of each foot) and the pelvis (a line between the ankle bones running across the foot). In this area are the reflexes for: parts of the digestive system, including the stomach, liver, gallbladder, and intestines; parts of the urinary system, including the kidneys and ureter tubes (which drain the kidneys); parts of the hormonal system, including the pancreas and the adrenal glands; and the spleen.*

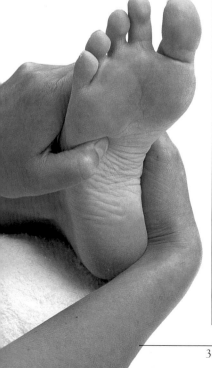

1 The reflex to the liver is found only on the right foot, in the area between diaphragm and waist level, in a triangular shape. The reflex to the gall bladder is found just below the liver reflex, and just above waist level.

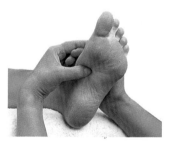

2 The reflex to the stomach can be found in the area between the diaphragm and the waist level, and overlaps the reflex to the pancreas.

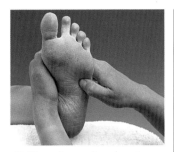

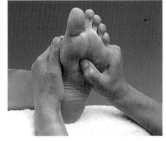

3 The reflex to the spleen is found only in the left foot, and to the outer side of the area between diaphragm and waist level. The spleen is responsible for filtering toxins and bacteria from the lymphatic system. It also produces antibodies.

4 The reflex to the solar plexus is just below diaphragm level on both feet. The solar plexus is a network of nerves with branches to all parts of the abdominal cavity; these reflex points are massaged to relieve stress, fright, anger, and nervousness.

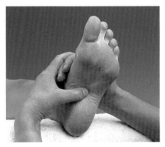

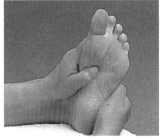

5 The reflex to the long small intestine is found in both feet, below waist level and above the pad of the heel, and is surrounded by the reflex to the large intestine, which starts on the outer side of the sole of the foot.

6 The reflex to the adrenal glands is just above waist level on top of the reflex to the kidneys on each foot.

The pelvis

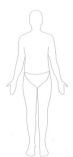

THE PELVIC AREA *of the body is represented on the foot just over and above the pad of the heel. The level of the pelvic floor on the foot runs in an imaginary line across the pad of the heel between the anklebones. Reflexes relating to areas of the pelvis are also found on the outer side of the foot.*

Reflexes for the following areas of the body appear in the pelvic area on the foot: the bladder, the reproductive glands, and the rectum. At the back of this area are the reflexes for the sciatic nerve, the sacro-iliac joint (where the sacrum of the spine joins with the ileum of the pelvis), and the pelvic muscles.

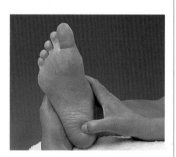

1 The sciatic nerve reflex is actually the nerve itself. This runs like a stirrup up both sides of the fleshy pad of the heel, and is therefore very sensitive.

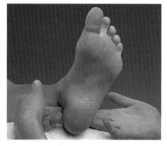

2 The reflex to the sciatic nerve also extends across the sides of the foot, and for a short distance up the back of the leg.

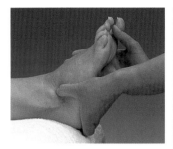

3 The reflex for the sacro-iliac joint at the side of the heel may be massaged during pregnancy if there is pain in the area.

DOREEN BAYLY

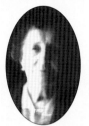

Doreen Bayly (1900–1979) deserves much credit for her endeavors to spread the interest in reflexology, because there was initially little enthusiasm for her work. Gradually her efforts were rewarded but she died just before the therapy received due acclaim.

The pelvic muscle reflex

The limbs

THE REFLEXES *for the limbs can be found down the outer side of the foot. The limbs that are located on the right side of the body are represented on the right foot, and the limbs on the left side of the body are represented on the left foot.*

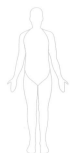

Shoulder reflex

1 The reflex to the shoulder is found at the base of the little toe on the sole of the foot, as well as on the top of both feet.

The left hand works the right shoulder reflex

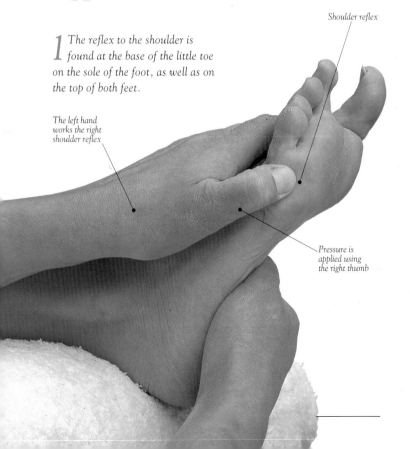

Pressure is applied using the right thumb

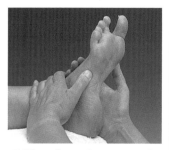

2 The reflex to the arm extends down from the shoulder area to the bony projection which appears about halfway down the outer side of the foot.

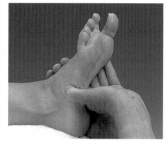

3 The reflex to the elbow is found over the bony projection about halfway down the outer side of the foot. Tennis elbow and Repetitive Strain Injury may be eased by addressing this reflex.

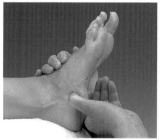

4 The reflex to the knee (and lower leg) is behind the bony projection on the outer side of the foot, extending to halfway toward the back of the heel in a half-moon-shaped area. The right knee is represented in the right foot and vice versa.

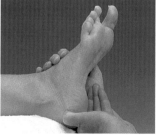

5 The reflex to the hip (and upper leg) is found extending from the knee area to the back of the heel in a half-moon-shaped area on the outer side of the foot. The right hip is represented in the right foot and the left hip in the same area of the left foot.

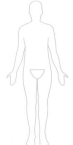

Reproductive organs and glands

IN THE FEMALE *the reproductive areas refer to the ovaries, Fallopian tubes, and uterus, while in the male they refer to the testes, vas deferens, seminal vesicles, prostate gland, urethra, and penis.*

The reflex areas to the reproductive systems are found on the sides of the feet and over the tops of the feet. In the male, the reflexes for the testes, vas deferens, seminal vesicles, prostate gland, urethra, and penis are found within this area on the foot. In the female, reflexes for the ovaries, uterus and Fallopian tubes are found within this area on the foot. Glands that affect both sexes will appear on the feet in men and women. The area on the sides of the feet is rather bony, and therefore lighter pressure should be used to treat these areas.

Ovary reflex in women or testes reflex in men

1 The reflex to the ovary in the female, and the testes in the male, can be found halfway between the outer ankle bone and the back of the heel.

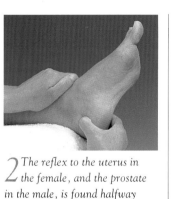

2 The reflex to the uterus in the female, and the prostate in the male, is found halfway between the inner ankle bone and the back of the heel. There is also a reflex to the uterus or prostate up the back of the leg for a short distance on either side of the Achilles tendon.

BELOW **Finger pressure can be used over the top of the foot to work the reflex to the reproductive area.**

3 The reflex to the Fallopian tubes in the female and the vas deferens in the male is found joining the two other reproductive areas over the top of the foot, passing just in front of the ankle bones. Treat each ovary and Fallopian tube on the appropriate foot; i.e., the left foot for the ovary and tube on the left side.

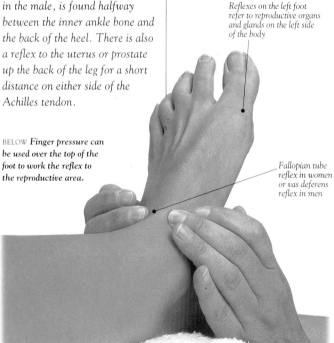

Reflexes on the left foot refer to reproductive organs and glands on the left side of the body

Fallopian tube reflex in women or vas deferens reflex in men

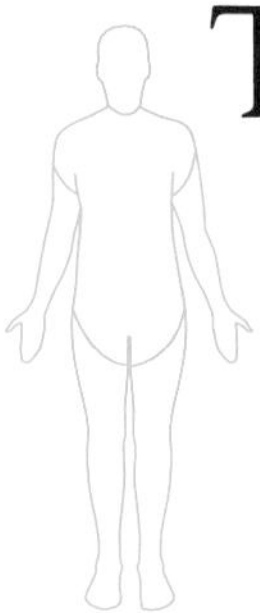

The lymphatic system

THE REFLEXES *to the lymphatic system are found on the top of the foot, extending down from the base of the toes to over and around the ankles. This area requires a lighter pressure than the sole of the foot.*

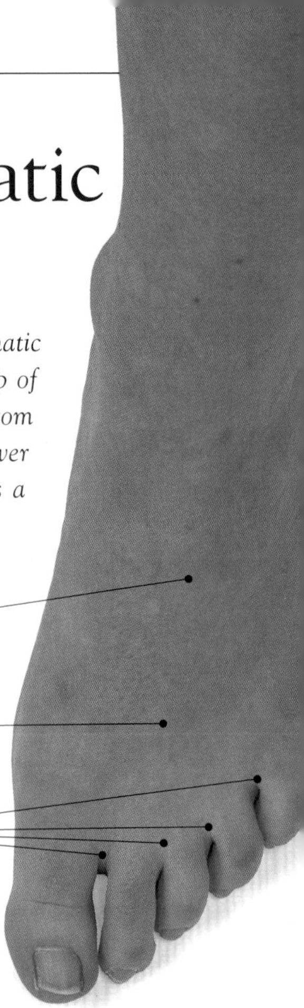

Abdominal lymphatics

Breast area

Upper lymph nodes

ABOVE *The lymphatic reflexes are found on the tops of both feet.*

The lymphatic system runs parallel to the circulatory system throughout the body, and is made up of lymph vessels, lymph nodes, and specific areas of lymphatic tissue. This system forms part of the "immune system."

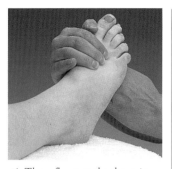

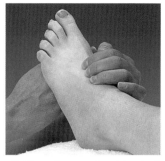

1 The reflexes to the thoracic lymphatics (the part of the immune system in the middle back) are below the toes on the top of the foot, to diaphragm level. This area includes the breast reflex.

2 The reflexes to the abdominal lymphatics continue down from the thoracic area to just above the ankle bones.

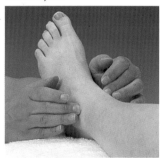

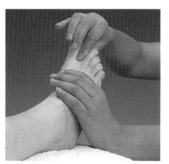

3 The reflexes to the lymphatics of the pelvis and groin are found over the tops of the ankles, and around the ankle bones. These areas might be stimulated for infections in the groin and pelvis region.

4 The reflex to lymph drainage is worked by pinching the area between the big toe and the second toe.

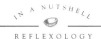
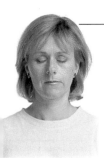

Foot exercises

WHEN ALL the reflex areas in the foot have been massaged, a few exercises are carried out. The exercises are intended to stretch the different areas and help you wind down. They include:

TOE ROTATION

1 Each toe is rotated in turn, by supporting the foot near the base of the toe with one hand, and holding the base of the toe between the thumb and fingers of the other hand.

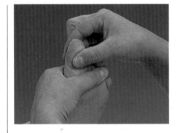

2 Rotate the toe around a few times in one direction, and then in the other.

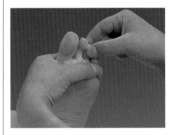

3 This is equivalent to rotating the neck, and helps loosen up the neck area. Where there is tightness in the neck, the toes – especially the big toes – may seem very stiff.

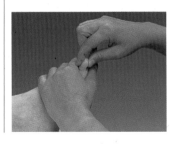

WRINGING THE FOOT

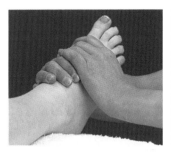

1 The hands are placed around the foot, with the thumbs underneath, and the fingers resting on the top of the foot. Pressure should be firm but should not cause pain.

2 Use the hands to wring the foot as you would a damp cloth. This action helps to spread the foot, and thus the body – rather like pulling the shoulders back, or taking a deep breath and stretching.

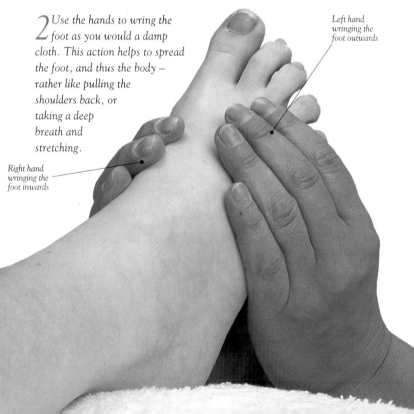

Left hand wringing the foot outwards

Right hand wringing the foot inwards

KNEADING THE FOOT

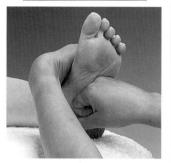

1 The flat surface of a clenched fist is pressed on the sole of the foot at diaphragm level, and the other hand is placed flat on the top of the foot.

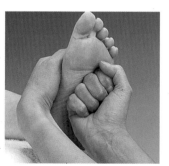

2 The hands are pressed against each other and rotated. This helps to relax the diaphragm, and so relax the whole body.

ROTATION OF THE ANKLE

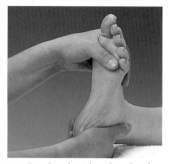

1 One hand is placed under the back of the heel, and the other hand supports the toes.

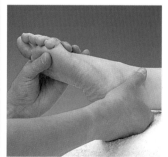

2 The ankle is rotated in one direction, and then the other. This helps to loosen any tightness in the ankle and the pelvic regions to help to ensure that energy flows unhindered through the body.

SOLAR PLEXUS BREATHING

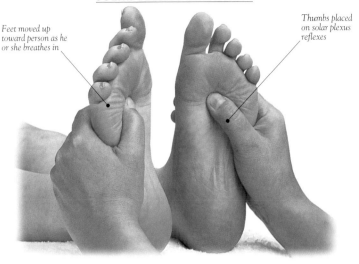

Feet moved up toward person as he or she breathes in

Thumbs placed on solar plexus reflexes

1 This exercise is done at the very end of the treatment session. The thumb is placed on the solar plexus reflex, right thumb on left foot, left thumb on right foot. As pressure is applied, the foot is eased up toward the person having treatment and he or she takes a deep breath in.

2 The breath is held, and then, as the patient breathes out, the pressure on the solar plexus reflex is released and the feet eased down away from the person.

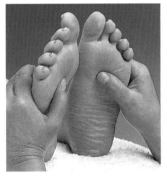

This is repeated three or four times and, apart from checking the breathing capacity of the patient, it makes a relaxing end to treatment.

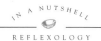

REFLEXOLOGY

Hand reflexes

ALL OF THE REFLEXES *found in the feet are also found in the hands, although the hands are not usually quite as sensitive to reflexology as the feet – probably because they are in constant use, and usually unprotected. Treatment is given to the hands in the same way as it is given to the feet, and the same techniques and order of treatment apply.*

As in the feet, the right hand will correspond to the right side of the body and the left hand to the left side of the body. Because the hands are smaller than the feet, the reflexes will be represented in smaller areas and are often more difficult to identify precisely.

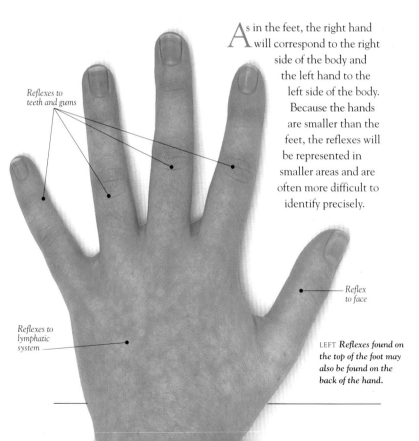

Reflexes to teeth and gums

Reflex to face

Reflexes to lymphatic system

LEFT **Reflexes found on the top of the foot may also be found on the back of the hand.**

However, some people will find that the reflex areas in their hands appear more sensitive than those in their feet.

The hands are treated in cases where the patient has very sensitive or ticklish feet, or where it is not possible to treat the feet due to injury or infection. The hands can also be useful for self-treatment if it is difficult to reach the feet.

The longitudinal zones that are present in the feet, and run through the body, also appear in the hands. The transverse zones are not as important in the hands as in the feet, and cannot be easily related to the skeleton of the hand.

A full treatment to the hands will take less time than a full treatment to the feet but can still be effective.

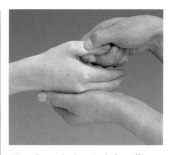

The reflex to the face, including all parts found within the face, is found on the back of the thumb below the nail.

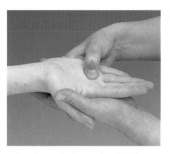

The reflex to the lung is found in the palm of the hand below the fingers, extending about one quarter of the way down the palm.

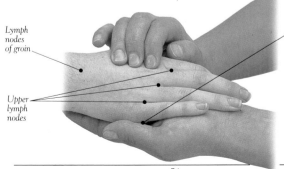

Lymph nodes of groin

Lymph nodes of axilla

Upper lymph nodes

LEFT *The reflexes to the lymphatic system are found on the back of the hand, working from the base of the fingers to the wrist.*

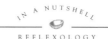
Reflexology at home

ALTHOUGH IT IS BEST *to receive treatment from a qualified practitioner, it may be possible to help certain ailments by working the reflex areas of your own feet or hands.*

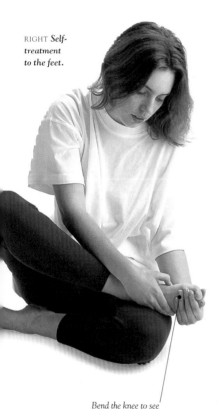

RIGHT **Self-treatment to the feet.**

WHEN NOT TO TREAT

In certain instances it is not appropriate to have reflexology treatment, or your practitioner will administer the treatment with extra care. In these cases, it is not recommended that you attempt to treat yourself. Do not try reflexology at home if any of the following conditions apply:

- acute infection
- diabetes
- epilepsy
- heart condition
- osteoporosis
- phlebitis or thrombosis
- pregnancy
- replacement surgery (e.g., hip replacement)

Bend the knee to see the sole of the foot

Common ailments

ALTHOUGH A FULL *treatment to all the reflex points is always given by a reflexologist, the reflexes which are particularly helpful to specific conditions are described below.*

ALLERGIES

• Reflexes to areas affected; e.g., nose, lungs, digestive tract, skin (*pp.35, 36–7*)
• Reflexes to adrenals, spleen (*p.37*)– to reduce oversensitivity.

ARTHRITIS

• Reflexes to the areas affected; e.g., hip, knee, shoulder, spine (*pp.40–41, 32–3*)
• Zone-related areas
• Reflexes to adrenals (*p.37*) – to reduce inflammation
• Reflexes to thyroid and parathyroid (*pp.34–5*) – for calcium balance
• Reflexes to intestines, kidneys (*p.37*) – to improve elimination
• Reflexes to pituitary (*p.30*) – for hormone balance
• Reflexes to solar plexus (*p.37*) – for relaxation, pain relief.

BACKACHE

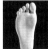

• Reflexes to affected areas on spine (*pp.32–3*)
• Reflexes to neck, sciatic nerve (*pp.30–31, 33*)– if affected
• Reflexes to adrenals (*p.37*)– to reduce inflammation
• Reflexes to solar plexus (*p.37*)– for relaxation, pain relief.

CHILBLAINS

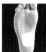

• Zone-related area – fingers for toes and vice versa (*pp.50–51*)
• Reflexes to heart (*p.35*)– to improve circulation
• Reflexes to intestines (*p.37*)– for good elimination
• Reflexes to upper spine and neck (*pp.32–3, 30*) – if fingers are affected.

COLD SORES

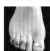

• Reflexes to areas affected: mouth, nose (*p.31*)
• Reflexes to lymphatic system (*pp.44–5*) – to help clear infection.

COLDS

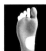

• Reflexes to areas affected: nose, sinuses (*p.31*)
• Reflexes to adrenals (*p.37*) – to reduce inflammation
• Reflexes to ileo-caecal valve and intestines (*p.37*) – for good elimination
• Reflexes to upper lymph nodes (*pp.44–5*) – to clear any infection.

CONSTIPATION

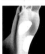

• Reflexes to areas affected: large intestine, rectum (*pp.37, 38–9*)
• Reflexes to small intestine, liver (*pp.36, 37*) – may be not functioning well
• Reflexes to lower spine (*pp.32–3*) – to ensure good nerve supply to intestines
• Reflexes to adrenals (*p.37*) – for good muscle tone to intestines
• Reflexes to solar plexus (*p.37*) – for relaxation.

COUGHS

• Reflexes to areas affected: lungs, throat (*p.35*)
• Reflexes to lymphatic system (*pp.44–5*) – to clear infection.

CYSTITIS

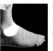

• Reflexes to areas affected; e.g., bladder, ureter tubes, kidneys (*pp.38, 36–7*)
• Reflexes to lymphatics (*pp.44–5*) – to clear infection
• Reflexes to adrenals (*p.37*) – to reduce inflammation.

DANDRUFF

• Reflexes to top of head (*p.30*) – for scalp
• Reflexes to adrenals (*p.37*) – to reduce inflammation
• Reflexes to intestines, liver, kidneys (*pp.36–7*) – to ensure good elimination.

DEPRESSION

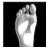

• Reflexes to areas affected: head (*pp.30–31*)
• Reflexes to solar plexus (*p.37*) – for relaxation
• Reflexes to adrenals (*p.37*) – to reduce stress
• Reflexes to pituitary and hormonal system (*p.30*) – to balance hormones.

DIARRHEA

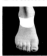

• Reflexes to areas affected: large intestine, rectum (pp.37, 38)
• Reflexes to small intestine, liver (pp.36–7) – may be not functioning well
• Reflexes to adrenals (p.37) – for good muscle tone to intestines and to reduce inflammation
• Reflexes to abdominal lymphatics (p.45) – to clear infection if present.

ECZEMA

• Reflexes to areas of skin affected; e.g., face, arm (pp.31, 41)
• Reflexes to adrenals (p.37) – to reduce inflammation and allergy reactions
• Reflexes to kidneys and intestines (p.37) – to ensure good elimination
• Reflexes to solar plexus (p.37) – for relaxation
• Reflexes to pituitary (p.30) – for hormonal balance
• Reflexes to lymphatics (pp.44–5) – to clear infection if present.

FLUID RETENTION

• Reflexes to areas affected (pp.41, 31); e.g., legs, eyes
• Reflexes to kidneys, ureter tubes, bladder (pp.36–7, 33) – for fluid elimination
• Reflexes to lymphatics (pp.44–5) – to clear excess fluid from tissues
• Reflexes to pituitary (p.30) – to ensure good kidney function
• Reflexes to heart (p.35) – for good circulation.

GLANDULAR FEVER

• Reflexes to areas affected; e.g., throat
• Reflexes to lymphatics, spleen, thymus (pp.44–5, 37) – to strength immune system and fight infection
• Reflexes to solar plexus (p.37) – for relaxation
• Reflexes to pituitary (p.30) – for hormonal balance.

GOUT

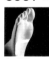

• Zone-related areas; e.g., thumb for big toe (pp.50–51)
• Reflexes to adrenals (p.37) – to reduce inflammation
• Reflexes to intestines, liver, kidneys (pp.36–7) – to encourage elimination
• Reflexes to solar plexus (p.37) – for relaxation, pain relief.

HAIR LOSS

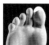

- Reflexes to areas affected: top of head (p.30) – for scalp
- Reflexes to adrenals (p.37) – to reduce stress
- Reflexes to solar plexus (p.37) – for relaxation
- Reflexes to pituitary (p.30) – for hormonal balance.

HANGOVER

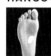

- Reflexes to areas affected; e.g., head (pp.30–31) for headaches
- Reflexes to liver (p.36) – to clear alcohol from system
- Reflexes to kidneys (p.37) – to encourage good elimination.

HAY FEVER

- Reflexes to areas affected: nose, throat, sinuses, eyes, head, face (pp.30–31)
- Reflexes to adrenals (p.37) – to reduce inflammation and allergy.

HEADACHES

- Reflexes to areas affected: head (pp.30–31)
- Reflexes to upper spine and neck (pp.30, pp.32–3) – to reduce tension
- Reflexes to solar plexus (p.37) – for relaxation
- Reflexes to eyes, sinuses, digestive tract, liver, hormonal glands (pp.31, 36–7) – which may be involved.

HEMORRHOIDS

- Reflexes to areas affected: rectum (pp.38–9)
- Reflexes to intestines (p.37) – to encourage good elimination.

INDIGESTION

- Reflexes to areas affected: stomach (p.36)
- Reflexes to esophagus, diaphragm (p.35) – closely involved
- Reflexes to solar plexus (p.37) – for relaxation.

INSOMNIA

- Reflexes to head areas (pp.30–31) – for relaxation
- Reflexes to solar plexus (p.37) – for relaxation
- Reflexes to adrenals (p.37) – to reduce stress
- Reflexes to areas relating to pain which may be causing problem; e.g., spine, teeth (pp.32–3, 31).

IRRITABLE BOWEL SYNDROME

- Reflexes to areas affected: intestines (p.37)
- Reflexes to adrenals (p.37) – to reduce inflammation and allergy
- Reflexes to solar plexus (p.37) – for relaxation.

ME 🐾

• Reflexes to areas affected; e.g., legs, arms, digestive system, head (pp.41, 36–7, 30–31)
• Reflexes to lymphatics, spleen (pp.44–5, 37) – to strengthen immune system and fight infection
• Reflexes to solar plexus (p.37) – for relaxation
• Reflexes to adrenals (p.37)– to reduce stress.

PERIOD PROBLEMS 🐾

• Reflexes to areas affected; e.g., ovaries, fallopian tubes, uterus, pituitary, thyroid, adrenals (pp.42–3, 30, 34, 37)
• Reflexes to solar plexus – for relaxation (p.37).

PMS 🐾

• Reflexes to areas affected: ovaries, fallopian tubes, uterus, pituitary, thyroid, adrenals (pp.42–3, 30, 34, 37)
• Reflexes to areas affected, as necessary; e.g., head, abdomen, breast, bladder, kidneys, intestines, face (pp.30–31, 36–7, 45, 38–9, 37)
• Reflexes to solar plexus (p.37) – for relaxation.

PSORIASIS 🐾

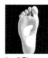

• Reflexes to areas of skin affected; e.g., face (p.31)
• Reflexes to adrenals (p.37) – to reduce inflammation and stress
• Reflexes to solar plexus (p.37) – for relaxation
• Reflexes to intestines, liver and kidneys (pp.36–7) – for elimination
• Reflexes to pituitary (p.30) – for hormonal balance.

SCIATICA 🐾

• Reflexes to areas affected: sciatic nerve and back of leg (pp.33, 38)
• Reflexes to spine (lumbar and sacral regions), sacro-iliac joints, pelvic muscles, knees, hips, or any area causing pain (pp.32–3, 39, 41)
• Reflexes to solar plexus – for relaxation (p.37).

STRESS 🐾

• Reflexes to areas where symptoms present; e.g., head for headaches (pp.30–31)
• Reflexes to adrenals (p.37) – to help reduce stress
• Reflexes to solar plexus (p.37) – for relaxation
• Reflexes to pituitary (p.30) – for hormonal balance.

THRUSH

• Reflexes to areas affected: uterus (includes vagina) (p.43)
• Reflexes to lymphatics (pp.44–5) – to clear infection
• Reflexes to adrenals (p.37) – to reduce inflammation.

THYROID IMBALANCE

• Reflexes to areas affected: thyroid (p.34)
• Reflexes to pituitary, adrenals, reproductive glands – for hormonal balance (pp.30, 37, 42–3)
• Reflexes to heart – if there are heart/circulatory problems (p.35)
• Reflexes to eyes – if they are affected with overactivity (p.31).

TINNITUS

• Reflexes to areas affected: ears (p.31)
• Reflexes to eustachian tube, sinuses (p.31) – may be involved
• Reflexes to upper spine, neck, side of head (pp.33, 30) – to release tension in area
• Reflexes to solar plexus (p.37) – for relaxation
• Reflexes to adrenals (p.37) – to reduce inflammation and stress.

VARICOSE VEINS

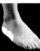

• Reflexes to area affected; e.g., leg through knee and hip reflexes (p.41)
• Reflexes to heart (p.35) – for good circulation
• Reflexes to adrenals (p.37) – to reduce inflammation
• Reflexes to intestines (p.37) – for good elimination.

Further reading

COMPLETE ILLUSTRATED GUIDE TO REFLEXOLOGY by *Inge Dougans* (Element Books, 1996)

REFLEXOLOGY FOR WOMEN by *Nicola Hall* (Thorsons, 1996)

REFLEXOLOGY: FOOT MASSAGE FOR TOTAL HEALTH by *Inge Dougans with Suzanne Ellis* (Element Books, 1992)

Useful addresses

The Bayly School of Reflexology
Monks Orchard
Whitbourne
Worcester WR6 5RB
Tel/Fax : 01886 821207
The Bayly School, established in 1978, has branches in London, Birmingham, Edinburgh, Leeds, Australia, Ireland, Japan, Kenya, Spain, and Switzerland.

Association of Reflexologists
27 Old Gloucester St
London
WC1N 3XX
Tel : 0990 673320

The Reflexology Association of America
4012 South Rainbow Boulevard
Box K585
Las Vegas
NV 89103-2059

The Reflexology Association of Australia
15 Kedumba Crescent
Turramurra 2074
New South Wales
Australia

The Reflexology Association of Canada (RAC)
11 Glen Cameron Road
Unit 4
Thornhill
Ontario L8T 4NB
Canada
Tel: 1 905 889 5900

The South African Reflexology Society
PO Box 201858
Durban North 4016
South Africa